Table of Contents

INTRODUCTION 2

DR. KAYLA MAI...4

CHAPTER 1 I Have Missing Teeth, Can I Get Implants? 7

CHAPTER 2...10
Other Options for a Missing Tooth.....................................10

CHAPTER 3...15
Sedation – How Many Kinds Do You Offer and Which One is Best for Me?...15

CHAPTER 4...20
Post-Operative Care: Recovery After Sedation and Healing Time After Treatment...20

CHAPTER 5...22
How Much Do Implants Cost? How Do I Pay For It? Are Your Fees Different Than Other Offices'? 22

CHAPTER 6 Do You Warrantee the Work That You Do?.25

CHAPTER 7 Will the Implants That You Put In My Mouth Look Nice and Natural?..29

CHAPTER 8...32
We Have Never Worked Together; Why Should I Trust You?...32

Dr. Kayla Mai's Thoughts About Our Doctors 34

Why choose our doctors?...34

CONCLUSION...47

INTRODUCTION

My name is Dr. Kayla Mai, the "Gorgeous Smile Designer" and "Romance Director." I create beautiful smiles and help strengthen people's relationships by taking care of them. I have been a dentist for about 15 years, and my passion is to help you achieve confidence and beauty. Whatever condition you are in right now, I would love to help you walk into a room and have everything in that space light up because you are just so beautiful. I want to help you feel amazing inside and out. I want you to land your dream job, to get promoted, and to fall in love all over again.

I love to uplift and elevate my patients in every way that I can, in every way that I know how. Through the art of dentistry and smile design, I want you to be able to eat your favorite foods without any dental pain and have that stunning smile that will change your life in ways that you never thought possible.

If you are over 50 years old and married, this book is for you. Maybe you look in the mirror and do not like what you see at all. The thought of seeing the dentist might keep you up at night, shivering and sweating because of your fears. Some of you have had to share these feelings with your partner; others have had to suffer alone. Because of your diminished self-esteem, loss of confidence, and pain, you are unable eat right, enjoy succulent kisses, smile at the camera, or go to social outings. I am here to help you change all of that. Soon, you will have a better, deeper, and more intimate relationship with your spouse or partner. You will smile again, make love again, and kiss again.

This book is also written for you if you are in need a lot of dental work and feel like you are the worst dental nightmare that any dentist could possibly see. You simply hate the dentist. You have been hurt, chastised, and made to feel horrible about your teeth and how you've neglected them. You want all your work done quickly, while you feel nothing. I promise to be with you the whole way and to work with you to end your fear and pain, so that you no longer have to disguise your face in public. Never will I judge you or talk down to you. It is not too late now…we can start somewhere. You will be surprised at what we can achieve in a short time once we put our hearts and souls into helping you through this exciting journey. Together, we will find a way to transform you into someone with beauty, grace, and confidence. We can do all this together without fear, anxiety or stress. Your transformation will happen quickly so that you can go back to your daily routine with a drop-dead gorgeous smile.

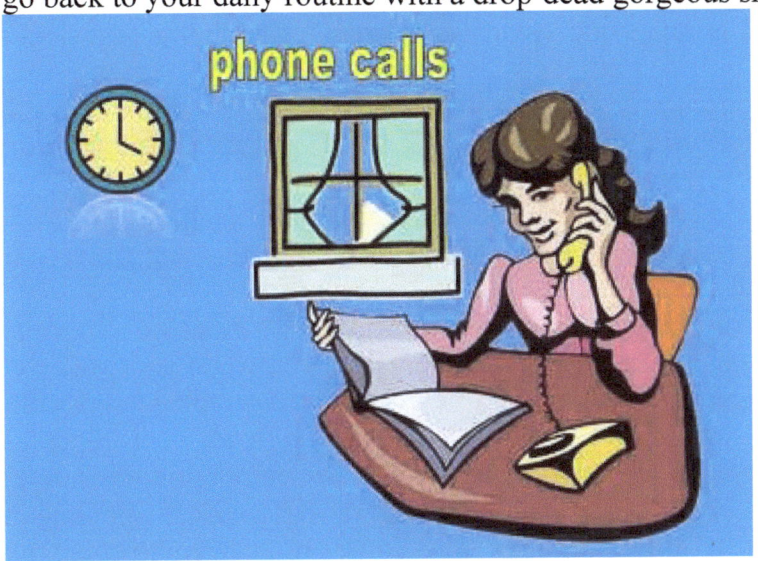

Call us at 702-475-8226 to schedule an appointment today. We have 20 slots each month open for a complimentary "Gorgeous Smile Consultation". Our place is extremely busy, so call now before space runs out! Mention code "Smile 2014".

DR. KAYLA MAI

Get to know your "Gorgeous Smile Designer" and "Romance Director"

I would like to tell you a little bit about my background. I came to the U.S. from Vietnam when I was about 8 years old. English is my second language. In this book, I write in simple words as though I am talking to you in person, without fancy language and technical terms. If we meet in person, you will recognize my voice having read this book.

I have 9 brothers and sisters, and parents who, to this day, do not speak English. I am the only person in my family with a formal education. I am a dentist today because of kindhearted people who selflessly helped me. I have experienced rejection, insecurity, and embarrassment because of my poverty-stricken background and horrible-looking teeth. I feel that, in life, I have "angels" that have guided me to this path. I feel that I was born to instill love, to make a difference, to care for you in ways that you have never been cared for before. Because I am so emotional, I have a "sixth" sense about you when you walk into our office. I would instinctively know if you felt scared, cold, hungry, or worried. I would also know if you were happy or excited. I have been helped, elevated, given opportunities in the darkest times of my life by strangers that expected nothing in return. My life now and my new smile are gifts from people that were at one time strangers.

In my early 20s, I was on my deathbed with meningitis, and I could not move for months. At that point, going to the bathroom or eating was impossible. Through life's miracles and the gifts of human "angels" surrounding me, I was able to live a normal life. I know deep down inside, it was true love that made me

4

heal, and the efforts of many that allow me to recover. I could not have done this healing on my own. Everyday, I look and I always see miracles like this happen in both small and big ways.

You may have a medical condition that leaves you feeling crippled, or you may have teeth that make you feel like you cannot face the public, just like how meningitis left me in my deathbed for quite some time. Whatever the seemingly horrible circumstance may be, it makes you human, and it creates an opportunity for you to run into "angels" that can help you. I have always believed that when we are faced with a physical, mental, or emotional condition that make us feel bad about ourselves, we also have an opportunity to meet someone amazing with a kind heart and a pure soul. If you are undergoing a hard time in your life because of your dental condition, I would like to be an "angel" guiding you.

I can relate to you from personal experience and will work with you at your comfort level in a high tech, yet calming environment. I notice that people hate going to the dentist and usually don't know which dentist to see. These people would prefer to give birth or even jump off a cliff rather than go get their teeth fixed! I see that there is a need for a relaxing, nurturing atmosphere where they can go to find comfort and friendship. Many do not go to the dentist because it is so uncomfortable and painful. We have changed all of that.

We aren't the cold, dark medical facility that you may imagine us to be. Rather, our office is a place that feels like your own home. In our clinic, you will smell baked cookies and will be pampered with blankets, pillows, TVs, iPods, and iPads. You will get plenty of personal attention and genuine care. Many of our guests say that coming to see us is a vacation from life, work, and stress. They just want to come here and lounge around. We have a high tech yet comfortable surrounding that nurtures growth, change, and beauty.

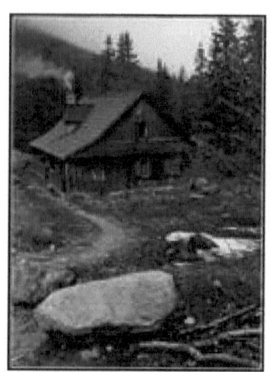

CHAPTER 1
I Have Missing Teeth. Can I Get Dental Implants?

I'm missing a tooth. How do I know I need a dental implant? What is a dental implant? Do I have to take it in and out?

Dental Implant

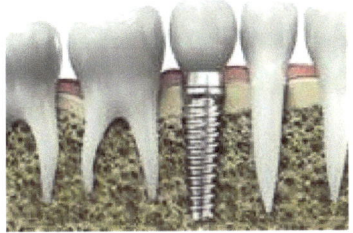

A dental implant is permanent: no glue, no wiggling in and out. It looks and feels like you were born with it – just like a natural tooth.

When you're missing a tooth, the best option out there is a dental implant. The reason why we recommend this most is because the dental implant feels like a miracle treatment, allowing you to have your new tooth and make it look as though you were born with it. It is the only treatment for a missing tooth that allows you to eat, drink, and feel as if you have our own tooth.

It is actually a very simple process. When you have a missing tooth, we place a false root (or post) where your tooth was, and link it to a false tooth that is the exact shape and size as the normal one.   It's just like your own tooth.

We do drill in a post inside your bone where there was a missing tooth. I only say that because people ask me this, and technically, you *would* see it on the X-ray, but you don't actually feel that it's there. So for instance, right now you have a lung and a heart. Do you walk around consciously thinking, "There's a lung and a heart in my body?" Probably not, right?

So, let me think, what else do you have? You have bones, right? You probably don't think about the bones in your leg, hand, or fingers. With the dental implant, the same applies. It's just something that sits there—you don't think about once it's in there.

The implant procedure

On TV, you are told that an implant takes one day. In reality, it takes about 6-12 months to complete the procedure. After that, you eat and smile normally. It is permanent.

Perhaps the most common questions are about whether the procedure hurts. Actually, many patients are surprised at how comfortable it is compared to what they were expecting. We are very gentle in our practice. We do a lot of extra things to make the process very, very simple. We even put lip balm on you. Patients are often surprised that they are not limping around in agony, as they might have imagined. Although there may be slight discomfort or soreness and swelling during a short recovery period, your life will quickly return back to normal.

Knowing how much fear and anxiety you may have, knowing how much you hate going to the dentist, we are very kind to you and treat both your face and mouth with care. We have certain ways to make this process more comfortable than a typical surgery. In fact, most people don't even notice a difference after it is done. Patients often tell me how surprised they are at how easy it all is. They seemed to think that the surgery is like giving birth or donating an organ...it is not like that at all.

What are implant- supported dentures?

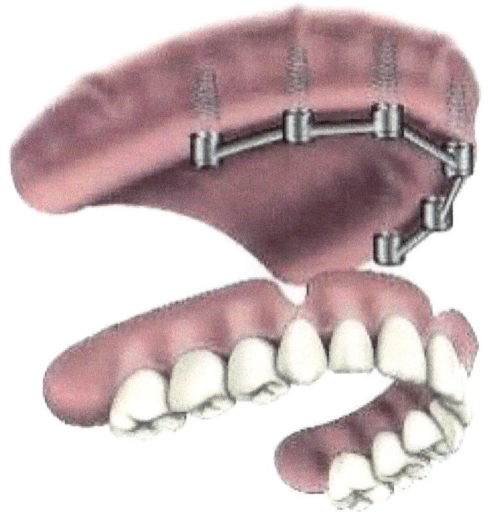

Full dentures are made when you have no teeth left either on the top or bottom arch.

Having implants in your mouth when you lose all your teeth will allow you to keep the bone in place. If you don't have any natural healthy teeth or implants, your bone will quickly deteriorate and your face gets sunken in. Wherever the implants are placed, bone is preserved. You look younger and more attractive when your face is properly contoured!

Implant dentures allow you to function so that there is no movement when you speak, eat or kiss. Imagine teeth flying out of your mouth when you are at a high school reunion or when you are kissing! Implant supported dentures allow your false teeth to be "locked" into place. You no longer need glue to keep your teeth in. Because there is no movement with implant-supported dentures you can eat and go about your daily routine.

CHAPTER 2
Other Options for a Missing Tooth

Bridge

A bridge is permanent, with three parts connected together into one piece
This is the second best choice for a single missing tooth
You can eat with this

Before implants, the bridge was the only way to replace a missing tooth. It is the second best option when implants do not work out. Most cases of implant failures result from not having enough supporting bone or the body rejecting the implant and pushing it out of your body. Another reason may be gum disease you are not aware of and the implant is living in an unhealthy environment.

Let's just say I am planting a tree. This tree needs good soil and sunlight to grow. The tree is like your implant and the soil is your healthy gums and your supporting bone. If the grounds are infertile and there is no sunlight, then the tree dies. The "dying" tree is analogous with a failing implant. Severe gum disease is like the infertile ground. Implants need healthy gums and bone to thrive.

Let me explain what a bridge is to you in a way that makes sense in real life. You are crossing from one side of the river to the other. You have land on one side, water in the middle, and land on the other side, right? So, you're making a bridge to connect from one side to the other so that you don't fall in the river. Land on either side holds the bridge. The most stable parts are the anchors land on either side.

So, with a bridge for teeth, you have to cut the teeth on either side of the gap left by your missing tooth, and then you have to connect so it becomes three teeth: the one that you're missing and the ones next to it. In other words, to replace that missing tooth, you have to involve two other healthy teeth. This is why a dental implant is a better choice if that option is available. Also, because a bride is hard to maintain, the surrounding teeth that you take down may end up needing further work later on. When you bite down, it's not even. You bite down on the "river" part of the bridge. It keeps moving around even though you may not know it, and then it gets cavities and holes, and it rots a lot faster.

A bridge is like three teeth glued together in one piece. Although bridges are not the best option, there are tricks to on how maintain them. We will show you how this is done if you decide to pick this option.

Partial

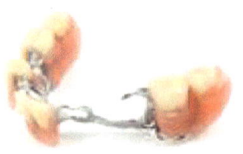 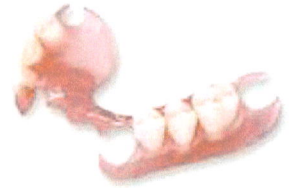

With a partial, you need to take it in and out at night
This is the 3rd best option for missing tooth/teeth.
Some people can wear this, others can't
Some people can eat with it, others can't
The good news is—it keeps the spaces open and prevents teeth
from shifting around

A partial is a fake piece of acrylic or metal with false teeth and gums all in one piece. It replaces all the missing teeth in the arch. You have a top arch and a bottom arch. You have some natural teeth and you have some false teeth. The false teeth dangle on the remaining teeth that you have. People complain that it is too big. It's a plastic or metal piece with teeth on the top that you take in and out. If you dangle something around the neighboring teeth for long enough, you're going to be wiggling those teeth around as well. Eventually, the support teeth (meaning your existing teeth that are still there) will need additional dental work.

In my experience, I would say that half of the people who want partials pay for them, but don't really wear them.

It is a good option if you are on a budget and willing to try to eat and smile with it. Knowing how difficult it is to like and wear a partial, we use the best material in the market to make it as comfortable as possible.

Can I replace a bridge with an implant if I already have a bridge?

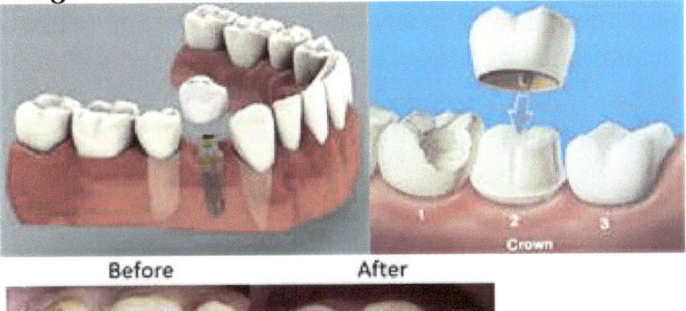

Before   After

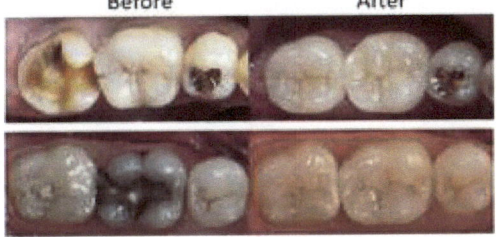

Replacing a bridge with an implant is an excellent idea, because when you put the implant where there is a missing tooth, you take the pressure off of the neighboring teeth. The empty space is now filled in with the dental implant. As long as there is enough bone to put the implant there, we are in good shape.

In other words, say I'm really heavy in the middle, with two people carrying me at both ends. Now I've gotten so heavy that my butt is hanging on the floor. I'd need a third and fourth person to hold me up. This concept works quite well for teeth, and implants are very stable and as easy to clean as your own teeth.

There are a few cases in which a bridge is a good option, but you should definitely get an implant if you qualify, because it's like a miracle. You have another tooth that's like your own. You smile normally. It's beautiful. You're able to eat like normal.

Overall, an implant is just a better overall choice, as it's conservative for the patient and is a more permanent option. This is what we recommend whenever we can for our patients who are good candidates.

The rest of this book will explain this process.

CHAPTER 3
Sedation – How Many Kinds Do You Offer and Which One is Best for Me?

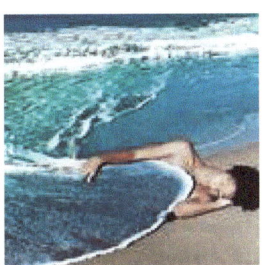

Sedation is for those of you that have high fear and anxiety, have not been able to get numb in the past, have a strong gag reflex, or have such a busy schedule that you want all the work done in 1-2 visits. If you pick sedation, you are telling us that you definitely don't want to remember the needle or what was being done. This is what we are most often told for those who want sedation: "I don't want to know, don't want to feel anything."

Are dental implants something that's done under local anesthesia, or is the patient sedated?

We can decide together if you would like to be completely alert and awake for your implant appointment, or be sedated and take a nap so that you are comfortable. We have found that over 90% of our patients like sedation, whether they are getting one implant or their whole mouth fixed with dental implants. They prefer taking a nap and not knowing what's going on. It is their time off from life and all the hectic events going on out there.

What types of sedation do you provide?

---Nitrous Oxide

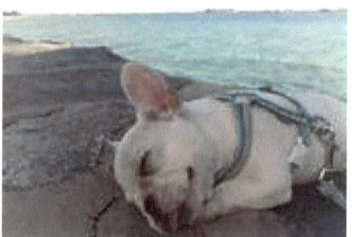

Nitrous is commonly known as laughing gas. We recommend this if you have one or two implants done in a region that's easy to get numb. You have very little anxiety and you are fine going to the dentist. This takes the edge off—you can drive to the office and you will be fine driving home. It goes through your body and wears off very quickly.

This is very light, and is for taking the edge off only for very short appointments. For this reason, it is not recommended for moderate to long surgeries. If you want to be awake and alert when you leave, pick this one.

---Relaxation/ Anxiolysis

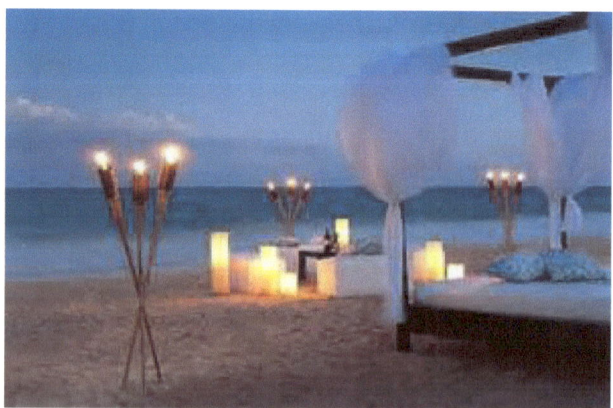

For this one, we give you a few pills to relax you. For some people, they get sleepy; for others, it has little or no effect.

---Deep Relaxation/Oral Sedation

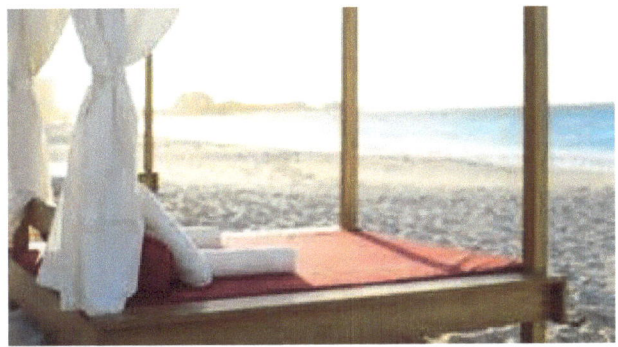

This is considered conscious, meaning that you can breathe on your own without life support.

You take pills and we give you a little bit more medication at a time until you are comfortable and you hardly care about receiving treatment. You will be monitored with a machine for your oxygen level and blood pressure. It works better than relaxation. For some people, it works great. For others, it is not enough.

So, if you're one of those people that have had a bad experience—you gag, you hate the dentist, you'd prefer to climb the highest mountain in the world, you'd prefer to give birth to ten kids in a row instead of go to the dentist! I would recommend sedation. You take a nice, restful nap. When you wake up the work is done.

IV Sedation

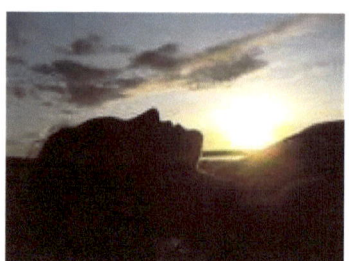

If you are worried about IV needles at this point and avoid IV sedation, we completely understand. Just know that we can give you something to drink to relax you before we put the IV in. The treatment is more gentle and kind this way.

This is also a conscious sedation because you don't need life support. You can breathe, talk, and respond to simple commands. You won't remember much and will not care what is going on. This is our patients' absolute favorite!

This is the best route if you want as much work done as possible. Of all the sedation procedures that we perform, this works the best. We give you medicine through an IV line that goes from your arm or hand that flows into your body.

Sometimes we put medicine in your arm muscle too. Like when you get a flu shot at your medical doctor's place.

Am I able to drive home after that?

With sedation, you need a driver and then you need time off from work. It's just like a little vacation, very simple.

For time off from work, what is the recovery time once I have this implant done?

If you do sedation, I tell my patients to take the next 24 hours off. If you need your whole mouth done in one visit or have many surgeries in one appointment, then just make your work schedule flexible enough to allow you to

General Anesthesia

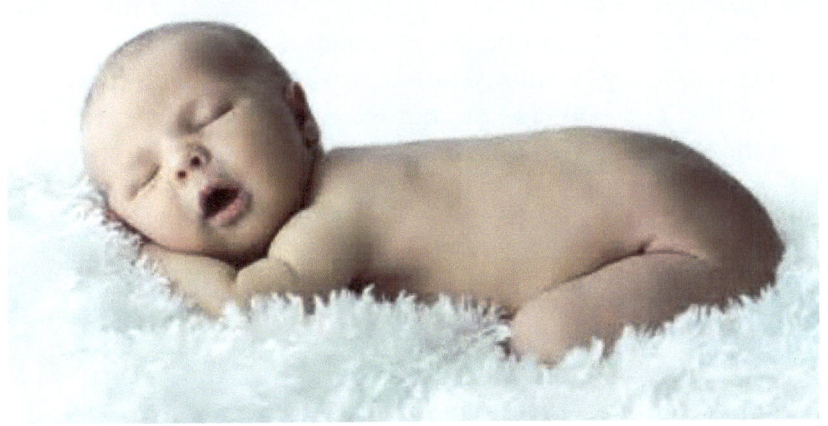

You are completely out and may be intubated. We do this on adults and children 18 months and up. The procedure is reserved for children, family members and adults that say, " I want to be completely knocked out!" According to anesthesiologist, it is safer to get this done than to drive to our office. General anesthesia is less risky than driving to Las Vegas! We do a thorough review of your health history. We coordinate your schedule with our anesthesiologist to make all this happen! You will really love this! What a dream come true!

CHAPTER 4
Post-Operative Care: Recovery After Sedation and Healing Time After Treatment

How long does it take to remove any stitches or sutures?

Typically with implant surgery, you have stitches and that's one of the things that'll drive you nuts. Usually within a month or so, we take it out or it falls off on its own. You're not going to like it, but remember for anything worth it in life, there's a little bit of something. I'm going to be honest about that. If I have a piece of broccoli hanging down my throat, it will really bother me. So, we know that this bothers you, but we have to keep it there. It's one of the things that you have to deal with. But we're there for you the whole time.

When you come in, we're going to prepare all your medication (antibiotics and pain meds) and go through that with you. We always prepare you for everything.

Why do I need to take all the antibiotics?

If you're given the antibiotics, you need to take them all because if you don't, they're not going to work. A lot of people stop after only a couple of days. This defeats the purpose. Please take all of them so that your body is not desensitized; it works really well. Just follow the instructions you're given for the medication and you'll do great.

How soon before I can chew?

With the implant, you need to wait for healing in that area, so typical implants take anywhere from six months to a year. It's like giving birth to a child; you have to wait for healing. That is the downside of the implant. But if you want something quality, that's what makes it a miracle treatment. You have to wait because implants have a few parts. You have the bottom underneath inside that you can't see and the top that you can see, which is what you see when you smile. You can see the white crown or the top of your tooth, and then there's a connecting part.

So that takes about six months to a year more or less, and it's individually catered to the healing of a patient.

So what do I do in the meantime? Say I just had an implant done. Can I still chew food on, let's say, the left side of my mouth where the implant was done?

You can chew around the implant just like with any surgery in life. You want to avoid the area for a while, but not for too long. By the time you're used to it, you have a tooth already. And if your smile is in the smile zone, we actually make you something there. We live in Las Vegas right now. It's an entertainment city. We do implants in a lot of smile areas, so whatever you do when you come out of our office, you're not going to walk out feeling ugly. You're going to walk out pretty attractive. We'll find a way to make it happen.

Take the day off for treatment, and make the next few days off in case you need it. For some of us, one or two days is plenty of time off. It's really rare that you would need weeks and months off, but you do deserve some time off!

Will I remember anything about the procedure?

Under sedation, you may remember my hair sticking up, or me tucking you into bed as we give you blankets, pillows, and things. Our patients tell me they don't remember the dental procedure at all. It's very, very comfortable. You must be so surprised reading this.

CHAPTER 5
How Much Do Implants Cost? How Do I Pay For It? Are Your Fees Different Than Other Offices'?

In our office, we would like to be up front and honest about money, so that you can plan appropriately without stress. It is an honest form of communication.

How much is a typical implant?

Typically, an implant is estimated at $2,000 to $4,000 per implant. You might have heard on TV that $100 to $200 per implant. I really don't know where those figures come from, but I will tell you that whatever we buy to start the work is a lot more than that. We do want to use products that last for many years. This is sitting in your body. You don't want something cheap when it needs to have the potential for life-long results. Do you want a cheap smile? Do you want a cheap heart or cheap lungs? This is not where you want to go cheap.

If I have people sending ads for cheap dental materials and services, I don't even look at them. So, whatever we have to do, whatever material we have to buy to make it last and to make it work, we do it. We don't cut corners to save money. We don't know what the fee is until you come in to see us, but anywhere from $2,000 to $4,000 per implant is within the range, more or less. But once you meet us, we'll tell you the exact fee so that there are no surprises.

At $2,000 to $4,000 per tooth, does that get covered by insurance?

Often when you call your insurance, they'll say they cover it. In reality, most of the time, they don't. So, don't feel like they're lying to you or that we're lying to you. We have done this for a long time, and we know more about your dental insurance than the insurance people often do. If they tell you that they cover it, we don't know until they actually pay it, and we've seen maybe a handful of insurances that pay in the over ten years that we've practiced. We normally just go through the whole fee with you, and find a way to settle a payment plan to make it affordable for you. But I will tell you that our happiest patients are implant patients. They're really happy because imagine you can't eat anything with this big gap in your mouth. Your teeth are moving around and then suddenly—voila! There's a tooth!

Do you pre-verify with the insurance company before anything else is done?

Typically for implants, we assume they don't pay. Hopefully, as time goes in, more insurance will cover this procedure. A few do pay, and we know which ones those are. But we do help you set up the payment plan. We make all of the financial arrangements in advance, so we can then just go ahead and reserve the time with the doctor.

Do you accept credit?

CareCredit®

Yes, and we have a payment plan available through a company called Care Credit, which patients can apply for online in the office in order to pay for treatment. It takes actually about three minutes to get approved. You can go to carecredit.com for more information. We also have our own office payment plan. The key is that knowing this is what you want; we'll find a way to help you. We have actually found that families, friends, and neighbors sometimes help you with the payment as well if they really care about you and you really want this. I've seen it happen often. With some of my patients who have no money, others will come to help them.

What if I have bad credit?

If you have bad credit, we do offer an in-office payment plan. You will need a down payment and monthly payments that we can preset with your checking or savings account.

Your family and friends from anywhere in the United States can always call in to make a payment for you on their credit card. This only takes a few minutes on the phone. At least 50% of our guests need help from loved ones.

CHAPTER 6
Do You Warrantee the Work That You Do?

In our office, we have a warrantee form that spells out exactly what the conditions are for the warrantee. We want everything to last for multiple years. We don't want you back with problems. If you do return for help, we are there to help you every step of the way.

We like the implants we offer to last as close to a lifetime as possible. We do not offer a lifetime warranty, but we've had very few failures and the failures are usually something that we could foresee, which we would tell you ahead of time. Implants rely on the foundation, so you want to keep up your cleanings so that the implants have a healthy environment in which to live.

There are a few cases where, for instance, if you're driving on an incredibly rainy day, you may run into a car accident more often. So, we have cases where we feel like it's not going to work, it may fail, just like anything in medicine, and we would tell you ahead of time so that you know. If we offer the option of a dental implant, it is a compliment to you that your mouth is in good enough condition.

What happens if I have an implant done and years from now something cracks, falls out, or whatnot?

That is not likely, but if it did, you'd just come back and see us. We'd take care of you. The conditions are on the warrantee form.

Are there cases in which implants fail?

Yes. Not often, but the cases where implants fail is because of a foundation that is not strong. The foundation is the bone and gums that your teeth sit in. You have to make sure that any gum disease or concerns are handled at the same time or prior to committing yourself to implant care. You may also have health concerns; if so, please discuss your health with us. There are a few conditions that may affect healing. Also, it can be that while you're recovering, you may eat potato chips or smoke too much, which opens up the wound. There are definitely things you can do to minimize that. Is it 100%? No. There's no guarantee for lifetime longevity, but we don't recommend it to you unless we feel that it's going to help you. And we treat you just like our own families. So if I wasn't going to do it to my brother, sister, or husband, I wouldn't recommend it to you.

Do I have to get clearance from my doctor before I have this done?

There are cases where you need to do that and when you come in, we'll let you know if you need it. We've had to turn down very few patients with certain conditions because they weren't able to do it. So, if our doctor or myself recommends the treatment to you, just know that it's appropriate for you. If we need a medical release, let's just say you have a ton of medical conditions and you're at risk, we normally have you walk the medical release to your doctor so that we can have it back on time. Faxes tend to get lost and there are delays beyond our control. Sometimes you're here, you're ready to do the surgery, and the medical release is not here. In our office, we have systems to make everything efficient and it's proven to work.

Do I need to be on or off any meds before I have the implant done?

We'll review that with you when you come in because our treatment and care is customized to you. It's not a cookie-cutter practice. We care about you, so we look at each individual person. We'll look at what you are currently taking and review it with you. One piece of advice—don't stop anything you're currently prescribed until we tell you to do so. The most common condition that need medical release are blood thinners (like Coumadin or Warfarin), pregnancy, COPD.

There are also very few medical conditions, but don't assume you need to be off of the drugs without verifying with us and then we'll verify with your medical doctor.

The key is to see us first and do not assume anything until we meet and thoroughly review your health history.

Are there any side effects with the implant?

Some people are sore for a while. I haven't had too many people complain about it. They compliment us more than they actually complain. As with any medical condition, we all heal differently.

Most would say, "Wow, that's amazing. I didn't realize how simple it was. Had I known it was that simple, I would've done it a lot sooner." And the ones who do complain, they normally have trouble with everything else in dentistry. If they have a paper cut, it may take 9 months instead of 2 days. We'll figure who those people are and we'll help them appropriately.

When will I have a tooth in place?

Normally within six to 12 months on average, you will get yoru beautiful smile! Simply put, you have the initial implant placement, the screw, that you can't see while under sedation.

Our patients claim that it is that simple. If you are worried, just know that it is a lot easier than you think.

Your next visit is in a few months. You come back for a checkup two minutes here, five minutes there. And then when you're done healing, we put the top part on it.

The procedure doesn't take one day?

Sometimes we can do it for you in one day, but because we've seen failure and we want to be set for the long-term, we do take our time when necessary. This time allows for healing. Throughout the process, we will make sure you have a temporary replacement, so that nobody else knows what is going on.

CHAPTER 7
Will the Implants That You Put In My Mouth Look Nice and Natural?

What is the tooth you put in made of?

These implant crowns are usually made out of porcelain. If there is metal substrate, we will make it beautiful so that people cannot tell. We only use high quality materials.

How do you match it to mine?

We try to match it to what you have. It should look beautiful and normal. Nobody should say, "Where'd you get that implant done?" If it's in the "smile zone", we try to place it in an area where it looks like it's growing out of you.

A lot of my patients think this is a miracle treatment just because of the simplicity. And I will tell you that if they have a whole bunch of missing teeth and they get an implant done, they always come back to get the rest done.

Will I be able to smile normally with an implant? What does it look like when you're done?

Yes, you should smile ear to ear. If you have a bridge in the smile zone, they don't look very natural for the most part. This heavily depends your smile line. If you do a partial with metal in it, people can tell right away. When you do a dental implant, people can't tell.

How about with my speech? Will I be lisping or anything else like that?

You are the only one that will notice. We are our own worst critic. If you have it and are talking to me, I won't notice.

Also, while we're waiting for the six to 12 months, the temporary tooth replacement may make you lisp a little bit, but not enough for you to worry about. And back to our question about one-day implant dentistry, that can be done in very few cases. So when you see commercials on TV, it kind of blows up the reality of things.

In real life, if you think about it, every surgery requires healing time. Once in a while, there's a one-visit implant case. It's just so rare that I don't want you to think that you can get that done and if you are, I'll let you know who you are.

But at our office, we are honest and tell you upfront what you can go through. It's a different approach because if I care about you and love you, I don't want to give you a false sense of what's happening. I'd rather tell you about the bad things that can happen; we prefer to behave that way because that's how we grow, and our patients love us because we're like that.

How will I look with my implant?

An implant looks very normal, and very beautiful. When done properly, nobody can tell that it was not originally a part of the teeth that are there—it's not going to look fake; you're going to love it.

What about tooth whitening?

It's important to note that you can't whiten the implant, so when you come to our office, we do an interview to see what your goals are and then we make sure that everything is in harmony with your face, as you definitely don't want to have one white tooth in the middle.

You also wouldn't want three white teeth in the middle with the rest black. So we match up everything to make sure that it will look natural. Like I said, nobody should look at you and say, "Oh, what a beautiful tooth."

We put the implant in after you decide what shade you like, and some people actually do other stuff like veneers, which are among the other services that we provide. We wouldn't harm the teeth; our goal is to make you look your best.

This way, you'll be able to find jobs, kiss, date, and have an amazing relationship with your family, friends, and partner. We have found that dental implants are one of those things that make people very confident.

Unfortunately, if the partial is loose, then it may fly off when you kiss or eat. With the implant, when you kiss, it does not move. You do not even have to think about it being in your mouth.

CHAPTER 8
We Have Never Worked Together; Why Should I Trust You?

Why should I choose you?

We built the office the way that you would like it. Everything we do, we have your best interest in mind. We believe customer service is about putting you first.

We are a highly professional dental team that truly cares for each and every patient that we see. We view the relationship as a marriage, so we do not take in every patient that walks in the door. You are selective about where you go, and we are selective on who we see in our office, and who should go to another dentist. Once we accept you as a patient, we take every measure to give you the very best. Our doctors have some specialized training above and beyond dental school. Under one roof, you can get a lot of dental work done without traveling to different offices. We do sedation and we have special technology that would allow you to get that dazzling smile quickly.

Our dental team and assistants at the front desk have a deep passion for serving you. We are all here for you as if you are our won family. We screen our team carefully, as we have thousands of applicants for each position offered. We have carefully selected people who are naturally caring so that you can experience only the best. We definitely do not hire people to work here because it's just a job; there's got to be passion and care involved. With everything that we do, we ask the question, "If this was me, what would I do?"

There is no pressure to "buy" in our nurturing environment. We find that you make the best choices when you are given the freedom to choose in ways that are comfortable for you. It is our duty to educate you because we are the experts. You will not know what is best for you until we tell you. We take the time without wasting time. In other words, we are busy and efficient, but we will make sure that there is no "rush". If you need someone to listen or you need time put aside to focus on your wishes and needs, we will take the time. If you are crying, your best friend would comfort and take the time to listen, correct? We will be that way with you once we accept you as a patient.

If you do not belong in our office, we will let you know. If you feel that we are not a good fit, we do need to know as soon as possible. Once we start the relationship, we will nurture it.

Our doctors and team would not propose treatment to you if we wouldn't do the treatment ourselves. That is the philosophy in our office—we want to help you keep your teeth and gums healthy for life so that when you progress into old age, you can eat, chew, and smile with confidence.

If you were my brother, my sister, husband, or child, I would recommend the same thing. It's a hard society to live in nowadays. We want to be that place where you do not have to worry about trust.

I treat your smile, your emotions, and all of your concerns as though they are my own.

Dr. Kayla Mai's Thoughts About Our Doctors
Why choose our doctors?

I'm Dr. Kayla Mai, and I have handpicked our doctors especially for you. They will all take care of you as though they love you more than anyone else. They will treat you like a husband, wife, brother, or sister.

Throughout this chapter, you will meet four of our amazing doctors: Dr. A Lamancusa, Dr. A Roberts, and Dr. W Liu, and our anesthesiologist, Dr. Amanda Okundaye. These doctors are very honest and genuine, and you can trust them completely with your dental needs. They will communicate clearly with you on how they can help you. You have come to the right place. If you need a transformation to be able to date again, to land a new job, to fall in love again when you might have fallen out of love because you couldn't be physically close due to your smile or any other issues, you've come to the right place. If you have teeth "flopping around" that do not stay in place and you're really sick of it, you have come to the right place. If you just want people that you can trust completely and to be in a wonderful dental home where you feel so welcome, you feel there's so much kindness and care around, you've also come to the right place. You can see any of our doctors; we all have the same practice philosophy: keeping your teeth and your gums healthy for life - giving you that beautiful smile that's going to make the room light up when you walk in, helping you transform your life in the most positive way.

Our doctors have a lot of hobbies and interests. They have families and loved ones. However, when they do come into our office, they are focused on you. There is nothing and no one more important. You're going to feel so special in their hands. So I have personally picked Dr. Lamancusa, Dr. Roberts, Dr. Liu and Dr. Amanda to make sure that you are very, very comfortable, and I look forward to you coming in to see us. You

34

can go ahead and give us a call at 702-475-8226. We are a very busy dental practice. This month we're offering 20 complimentary consultations and smile designs. Call us today!

Dr. A Roberts

Words from Dr. Kayla Mai about Dr. Roberts:

I specially selected Dr. Roberts to join our team at Hi-Tech Dental Care. When we had an opening for a dentist a few years ago there were many applicants and Dr. Roberts stood out. People in the office tell me he's very handsome and clean cut; they're quite attracted to him. You know, you meet those doctors who can seem dirty, but he's extremely clean. There's something so perfect about him as a person. Dr. Roberts goes to church, and volunteers often. He shows up to every single volunteer event that we take a part in. He teaches kids about the Mormon religion, volunteers on Sundays, and his life is dedicated to service. That is just so amazing to me; instead of going out and drinking or wasting time, he spends his time teaching people about God. In the office, he educates people and then puts his heart and soul in the work that he does and is also a very honest person. So a combination of a good-looking dentist, who is highly ethical, cares about you, and is dedicated to service, I think to me is an outstanding find to us and we are so lucky to have him. I hope that you enjoy his company because you're going to really love all the work that he does and you're going to love him as a person. He takes great pride in his work and our patients are pleased with the results. In one instance, within a day, a wife fell in love with her husband all over again after receiving dental work from Dr. Roberts.

From Dr. Roberts about a patient:

> "When I met this patient, he told me, 'You know, my mouth's a wreck and I'm not quite sure what to do about it. I just want to be able to smile again.' I told him that we could definitely help him, and I told him that there were a few things we needed to start off with. We

focused on what he wanted to get done first. *It was about him, not about us. If we don't do what he wants, he won't feel like his needs are being met.* We definitely wanted him to feel encouraged because it's his mouth, and his dental health. Now, his teeth were a little bit crooked, and they were pretty broken down and had really dark spots, which was pretty unsightly for him. He didn't feel confident enough to smile, and he wanted to be able to, because he talks with people all day long. He works at a sandwich shop. When I first saw him, he was kind of talking with his lips down and would cover his hands with his mouth.

Well, we were able to get all of his work done in one visit so he went to sleep, and when he woke up, we showed him his teeth, and he was on the verge of tears at what he saw.

It was very fulfilling for me to see the effect that it had on him and the confidence it gave him. He was able to smile and he said, 'You know, these look exactly like my teeth used to look.'

And then, it was neat to hear from his wife. His wife had made the comment that she felt almost guilty, that she felt like she was cheating on him, because he looked like such like a new man!"

Dr. Roberts is from a large family—six siblings, and one is an identical twin brother who is also a dentist! Family is very important to Dr. Roberts, and he tries to spend as much time with his as he can. He has a beautiful wife and hopes to soon have a family of his own.

In his spare time, he has volunteered in Dentistry from the Heart for three years in a row and has donated at least $20,000 to $30,000 worth of free work in those three years.

You can come in and see Dr. Roberts for a complimentary consultation. Just call our office at 702-475-8226.

Dr. A Lamancusa

Words from Dr. Kayla Mai about Dr. Lamancusa:

When we invited Dr. Lamancusa, whom we call "Dr. Lam", we had a lot of applicants, and he really stood out. What is it about Dr. Lam that is so special? Have you had a friend, mom, dad, partner, husband, wife, or somebody that is always there for you? Someone you can reach out to who is always there? This is true about Dr. Lam. Whenever a team member needs something— our assistant, front desk (myself included), or a doctor gets sick, he is the first person to jump in and volunteer to just take over any job, do anything at any time. He reminds me of an old neighbor that cares about you, brings you soup when you're sick, and would take you to the hospital in the middle, in the middle of the night at 2:00 in the morning. You can just call him to go get your medicine. You come to him for comfort when you're feeling down. So from the moment I first talked to him, I realized he was beyond himself. I don't know how to explain that in words. I'm almost getting choked up and emotional now! I remember when one of our doctors was sick; I didn't even have to ask. Dr. Lam would just call in and say, "I'll be there," and he actually showed up and we hadn't even said "Yes" yet. When he found out that someone was accused of something and they were innocent, he said he would find them a judge or a lawyer. When a patient came in with crippling pain, he would actually do wonderful dentistry for them and then give him his cell number. This is after a whole day's worth of work with long hours where a patient would ask him to stay back because they would have to have their smile tomorrow. Besides having been a dentist for over 20 years, having such amazing experience, he works with his heart and soul. He cares about you as though he really loves you, and to me, that is a jewel of a person. He is a jewel of the practice. He just doesn't work on teeth; teeth are beside the point. Our doctors are very clinically excellent, but he does it with care and he does everything for you as though it's his own mouth and he loves you. I think that is very special about Dr. Lam. Sometimes he works long hours; anywhere from 9-12 hours a day. Our patients absolutely love having him in our office.

Dr. Lam is originally from Las Vegas—born and raised, went to high school there, and then went to college in Reno, grad school in Boston, and residency in Minneapolis. He comes from a family of doctors. His father is a retired medical physician, and his two brothers are both neurologists.

In his free time, Dr. Lam visits his lake house, which is a two-bedroom, two-bath trailer that he recently remodeled. There, he enjoys fishing (both traditional and spear fishing), water skiing, swimming, and just working on his tan. He also spends his free time cooking, practicing Kung-Fu, Philippino stick fighting, and sword fighting. He is currently single.

You can come in and see Dr. Lamancusa for a complimentary consultation. Just call our office at 702-475-8226.

Dr. W Liu

Words from Dr. Kayla Mai about Dr. Liu:

Of all of the doctors that we have in the office, I have known Dr. Liu the longest. It has been about twenty years now. Dr. Liu is extremely genuine and is going to tell you exactly what he sees and feels. He comes off as being very serious which causes him to not have the best first impression. On the outside, he is very conservative and does not smile very much, but on the inside he has reserved compassion for his patients and loved ones. He hardly has any wrinkles if you look! Dr. Liu cares very deeply about each and every one of his patients and wants to make sure that they get the best care possible. This stern personality allows him to be a very authentic and focused dentist. He is going to give you a solution to your problem and make sure that you are out of pain quickly. If you want a dentist who would never be dishonest with you and treats you like his brother or sister, then Dr. Liu is the doctor for you. I have noticed that once a patient has had a treatment done with Dr. Liu they always count on him and want to continue all of their future treatment with him.In my opinion, his work is of the highest quality. If you are looking for a dentist who is going to help turn your life around very quickly and conservatively – meaning that he does not do anything extra that you do not need – then definitely choose Dr. Liu.

He has done many implant cases and beautiful cosmetic work. He is very handy and creative. He is the one to come to if you would like to change your life and your smile and have the dental work last for many years to come—durable and lasting. His fans are mostly full mouth reconstructive case. Once you have him as a doctor, you will want him forever. For those of you that have had many dentists in the past, you will recognize his talent immediately because you are a "professional" patient. You have been around the block and you will just know.

Although reserved in his disposition, Dr. Liu has a talent of recognizing talent and showing appreciation. He has sent staff members to Hawaii for exemplary work, rewarded the team with the trip to Cancun for 5 days, and give out presents when they are due. He is the one the points out good efforts to me and make sure I see when someone is going the extra mile!

When thinking of Dr. Liu, I remember the phrase "the shallow murmur, but the deep are dumb". He does not make a lot of "noise", but all the work gets done efficiently, perfectly and quietly. He makes dentistry feel so easy and effortless.

Dr. Liu loves to mountain bike and do outdoor activities. He loves to go shooting at gun ranges and go golfing. When something breaks up at home, he would fix everything himself.

He's too busy to wash your car..but if he does, I challenge you to find any dirt or dust remaining. He does a better job than any premium car wash in the country! He has this talent for meticulous detail! He does dentistry with the same kind of care.

If you want a beautiful, healthy smile that is "forever lasting" with a doctor that has a deep concern about you, call Dr. Liu at 702-475-8226!

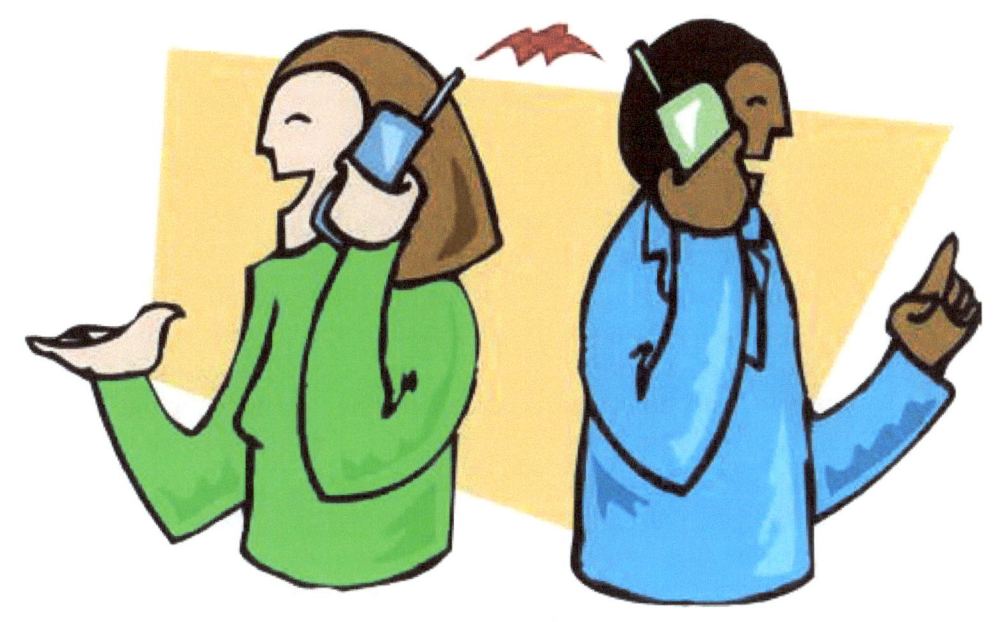

Dr. Okundaye - Anesthesiologist

Dr. Okundaye is our dental anesthesiologist. She usually goes by "Dr. Amanda", as most people are not sure how to say "Okundaye". Dr. Okundaye puts patients to sleep when they're having dental work done and can ensure that they are completely out...for patients aged 18 months to 100 years old! Sixty percent of her practice is treating children with special needs, specifically autistic and cerebral palsy children, and those who are really young. The other forty percent of her practice is the phobic adults or really medically compromised that otherwise wouldn't have a good experience at the dental office, which is where she comes in to help. Her number one job is to keep the patients safe. She also ensures that patients have all modalities of anesthesia so some patients can be conscious because of their health history and yet other patients can be completely asleep like children. It is most important to Dr. Okundaye to make a difference to the patients and for them to be happy and feel cared for.

Dental anesthesiologists attend dental school and then after dental school, they attend a dental anesthesia program for an additional three years, just like M.D. anesthesia residency students. Out of a thousand applicants, a typical school accepts only one resident per year, so a student has to really stand out, as Dr. Okundaye did and still does.

Dr. Okundaye is married with two children, ages one and five. Her husband is also a dentist, a prosthodontist for the VA clinic. In their free time, the Okundaye family enjoys sports and outdoor activities. Dr. Okundaye is passionate about her family and loves Sunday dinners.

Answers from Dr. Okundaye:

What are some of the mental disability conditions that you can handle in your dental experience?

"I have been so well trained at UCLA, so, a lot of conditions. It is a great school and our patient population is the combative, mentally compromised patient, so I'm very comfortable with understanding premedication, and understanding how some patients need a shot first. We have given mentally retarded patients a shot first in the car just to get them out and to get them in an office. So we have many different ways to help our patients who need behavior medication. With that being said, we treat the mentally challenged, the autistic, patients with Asperger's, cerebral palsy, any patient who has a mental disability or physical disability we really can work with."

Will dentists do minimal appointments because of sedation?

"With anesthesia, we can complete more work under anesthesia than alone. So what used to be a four-quadrant or four-appointment setting, we can do all, especially for children, four quadrants when a child is asleep in an hour and a half instead of four different appointments with oral sedation. It's also safe to not give a child, let's say, oral sedation four different times or bring a patient back four different times and families and, and patients themselves appreciate it because they're not taking off work and driving, so it's very cost effective."

Say I hate my smile and I hate the dentist, I have brown or black teeth, and I've been covering my face for the past 20 years. I can't even kiss my husband, I have bad breath. I feel really down, and I can't even go apply for a job. I've just been really down. I was really beautiful at one point when I was younger. I've been married for 30 years, and now I'm over 50. *What can you do for me to help someone like me, or is it too late?*

"First of all, it's never too late. The beauty of dentistry is that we have come so far and, and there's so many things that Dr. Mai and our other doctors can do for you. From my perspective and the anesthesia, I'm going to make you comfortable enough to where you can have your work done, not feel discomfort, not wake up very numb, and when you wake up and your temporaries are on, you're going to be a little loopy, but you are just going to be that much happier."

CONCLUSION

I am Dr. Kayla Mai, the "Gorgeous Smile Designer" and "Romance Director". What that means is that I can make you look and feel beautiful, which will improve your life in amazing ways. I can help you fall in love and stay in love. If you have a love life already, I can help strengthen your relationship by making you feel so stunning that your confidence and beauty will affect your love life in a positive way. I have a way of making people become better spouses, parents, significant others, friends, and lovers.

Today, we've talked about dental implants and how they are the best treatment for a missing tooth or teeth if you do qualify and why they are the best option over the other things we talked about, like a partial bridge or dentures that are removable. I highly recommend it because our patients who have dental implants are the happiest.

We talked about how this is a miracle treatment that you can get done under sedation if you choose, to where you hardly feel anything and don't even notice it's there, and heals in the timeframe of anywhere from six months to a year, more or less.

We also talked about ways of getting it financially, reviewing your health history, and seeing what concerns you have. We have to make sure that we address the issues.

We discussed the look of it and feel of it, the transformation, and the changes that it can do for you. Just so you know, after you get dental implants done, you can smile, so you go from covering your face to smiling from ear to ear. You're going to walk out feeling confident and beautiful with a very natural look. My patients tell me that they've been able to date and land good jobs afterward, and that they cannot believe that they can get this done. They didn't know that something like this can be done.

You're going to be dealing with a staff of very caring people and doctors you can trust who have a lot of experience. You don't have to worry about not being able to trust us because everybody that's in our office, I would be comfortable at this point to put my life in their hands. I ask myself if I would be comfortable putting my life in their hands when we hire someone. If you want to make an appointment, you can go ahead and give us a call. Our phone number is 702-475-8226. We are a very busy dental practice, so this month, the first 20 callers get a complimentary consultation, and also a smile design as well.

A smile design is basically a "snap smile design" where we take photos of you with digital imaging, and we can show you what a dental implant is going to look like before we even start. If you have a gap, we're going to show you what it looks like to close that gap with an actual tooth.

So go ahead and give us a call at 702-475-8226. We have only 20 spots available per month for this complimentary "Gorgeous Smile Design Consultation". Call us now! We are very busy and the appointments fill up quickly! Call to get that dream smile that will give you an amazing life! Mention code "Summer 2014". CALL TODAY! CALL US NOW!

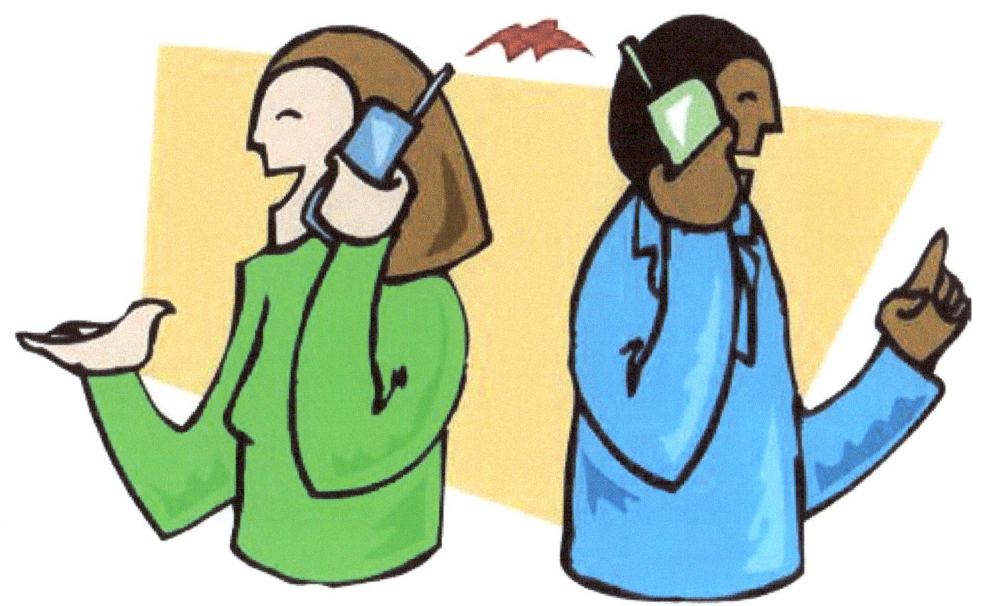